# Table of Contents

# Gluten-Free Lifestyle

By
Laura Dankof, MSN, ARNP, FNP-C

# Copyright & Disclaimer

# Do You Have a Sensitivity to Gluten?

There's a lot of information in the news about problems caused by gluten. There's a wide range of symptoms that can be caused by a gluten sensitivity or, even more seriously, a disease called celiac. Before we look at the symptoms, let's get to the basics of gluten. Gluten is actually a protein that's found in some grains. You'll find this protein in wheat, rye, and barley. It's not found in oats, but some oats get exposed to other grains during processing so it's possible to be exposed to it from eating them. There are also many flours that contain gluten and should be avoided.

Flours That Contain Gluten and Should be Avoided

- Wheat

- Rye

- Barley

- Graham Flour

- Bulgar

- Spelt

- Triticale

- Semolina

- Durum

- Farina

- Kamut

If you have a gluten sensitivity, eating foods high in gluten can be a miserable experience. You may find that you feel bloated and have digestive problems. You may also find that you have a hard time losing weight while some people lose weight because of malnutrition. When you are gluten intolerant, your body has a hard time absorbing the gluten protein that's found in wheat, barley, and rye. As you continue to eat these foods you may have a wide array of digestive problems – weight gain being one of them. This is because your sensitive to gluten is causing inflammation and poor nutrient absorption.

Don't believe it is possible to lose weight by going gluten-free. Try it for a month and see what happens. Not only may you lose weight, but likely you will feel better as well. **When you have gluten** intolerance you can feel fatigued and have headaches after eating grains that contain gluten. You may also experience gas, bloating, cramping, constipation or diarrhea. For some the symptom might be joint pain. Gluten intolerance can also lead to skin problems such as eczema. You may also have problems with irritability and even depression as a result of this sensitivity.

Celiac disease is a more serious reaction to gluten and is an autoimmune disease that can be very problematic. With this disease, eating food with gluten can cause terrible diarrhea, abdominal cramps, and other digestive problems. Celiac disease can be so serious that hospitalization and surgery are required.

If you've been having digestive problems, you may want to talk to your healthcare provider about celiac disease and get tested. Even if you don't have a serious form of celiac, you may find that you have a sensitivity to gluten. Beware however that the tests used to find celiac disease, are not finding gluten sensitivity.

While a gluten sensitivity once meant that you couldn't enjoy food, today's market provides many gluten-free food alternatives. You can easily find gluten-free bread, cookies, and cakes which wasn't possible twenty years ago. Often times these products are not nutritious. Look instead to eat whole, organic, unprocessed foods that are naturally gluten free.

If you suspect you have a gluten sensitivity, there's a simple way to determine if you're correct. Eating a gluten-free diet for several weeks should help you to feel better if you're suffering from the sensitivity. If eating gluten-free improves the way you feel, you probably have a intolerance. It often only takes two to four weeks to start feeling better.

If the change in diet doesn't have any effect on the symptoms you've been feeling, chances are you may not have a gluten sensitivity after all. You'll want to talk to your healthcare provider about some other causes for your symptoms. You may be sensitive to other foods, have small intestinal bacterial overgrowth, yeast overgrowth, or other reasons for your symptoms.

A gluten sensitivity can make life miserable with the wrong diet. But when you eat gluten-free foods you'll find that you can feel great and eliminate the miserable symptoms. Eliminating wheat, rye, and barley can make a major impact on your health and wellbeing. Be aware that many processed foods have hidden sources of gluten in them as well.

## Preparing to Transition to a Gluten-Free Diet

Going "cold turkey" into a gluten-free diet can be overwhelming. However, your bloated belly and constant discomfort may lead you to starting a gluten-free diet simply to get beyond the misery. The goal is to be able to free yourself from the discomfort and even debilitating symptoms of gluten intolerance, but you also need to prepare your mind and body as well as your loved ones for this transition. You'll need to talk with family members about your transition to a gluten-free lifestyle. Whether you should force your family into a similar diet is discussed in a chapter further along in this book.

To get your body prepared, consider doing a short detox program or fasting. Minimally, start to get into the gluten-free lifestyle by weaning yourself off your "must haves." Do you need to have a bagel every morning? Try substituting fresh fruit for the gluten loaded products.

At the grocery store, ask the manager where you can find gluten-free products. If he doesn't have any, be sure to tell him you'll be looking for an alternative grocer from which to purchase all your groceries until he starts stocking gluten-free products. Of course, make sure he understands that you'll tell your friends where you shop for gluten-free groceries, too! Thankfully, most grocery stores have a gluten-free section today. In fact, some stores even have dieticians on hand to help you. However, it is important to realize that foods labeled as being "gluten free" are not necessarily healthy. Some of them are high in carbs, calories and fat, and so will be a concern if you are trying to achieve a healthy weight. Furthermore, many of these foods are high on the glycemic index. Meaning they can spike your blood sugars, leading to greater insulin release.

This will sabotage your efforts to lose weight and lead to inflammation. The message here is that gluten free products are not necessarily healthy.

## What are Symptoms of Gluten Intolerance?

The most frequently heard complaint from people with gluten intolerance is that they suffer from digestive problems. Perhaps that is what led you to this resource you are reading now. Studies indicate that as much as fifteen percent of the United States population has trouble digesting gluten. However the number is probably actually much higher. You may very well be part of that statistic.

While many people don't know they have gluten problems until adulthood, you may wonder is gluten sensitivity limited to adults. In fact, gluten sensitivity can be experienced during childhood. As a parent, it's important to know what to look for with your child.

There are several symptoms that can suggest gluten intolerance. Each one by itself may not indicate a problem, but when there are several present you should talk with your healthcare provider about it. Just know that not all healthcare providers know how to look for gluten intolerance.

There are many symptoms which you might experience that could be related to a problem digesting gluten. People who have gluten intolerance are technically allergic to the gluten protein that's found in wheat, barley, and rye. You may feel badly after eating these things. When looking for gluten intolerance in your infant or toddler, you might notice he is not growing as fast as you'd expect. If it's related to gluten, it's because he can't absorb the nutrients from his food properly and it stunts his growth. It is important to point out there can be other reasons he is not growing faster or it may be normal to a point.

The most obvious symptoms with gluten intolerance are problems with diarrhea or constipation. While these two symptoms are at the opposite end of the spectrum, they're both possible if you have gluten intolerance. You may experience bloating and gas, too. You may have no digestive symptoms at all and be experiencing dry skin, eczema, easy bruising, headaches, mood swings, fatigue, and joint pain. This is largely due to the inflammation that it causes throughout the body. Depending on your body, you may experience only one or two of these symptoms while some people experience a multitude of them.

If you have long-term problems with gluten intolerance you may begin to either gain or lose weight without changing your diet very much. Weight loss is particularly common in people who have problems with frequent diarrhea.

When you go to your health care provider, your blood tests may reveal that you have a problem. Most of the time it won't and you and your healthcare provider falsely believe gluten is not an issue for you. Many people with gluten intolerance have low levels of nutrients in their blood. This is something that is rarely checked and insurance often will not cover the cost of a complete nutritional evaluation. For example, you may have a low amount of iron. This malnutrition is due to your body not being able to absorb nutrients.

Women who have gluten intolerance also tend to have more problems with their menstrual cycle. It may be irregular with no other explanation. Because of this they may even have problems with fertility and women who have gluten intolerance are also at greater risk for miscarriage.

There are behavioral conditions that are provoked by a gluten sensitivity such as, depression, irritability and constant fatigue. In fact, if you've recently been diagnosed with fibromyalgia, consider getting tested for celiac disease. Often these two disorders of misdiagnosed as the other. Regardless, try a gluten-free diet.

For a specific group of children who have autism, gluten can actually exacerbate the symptoms. Eating a gluten-free diet has been shown to improve the function of the brain in children who have autism – in some cases it has made vast improvements.

The theory behind this is since the adult human body has a hard time processing the wheat grains, children have greater difficulty. This has been linked to a condition referred to as "brain fog", which provokes symptoms of autism such as poor focus, irritability, and hyperactivity in children with autism. Removing gluten-based foods from the autistic child's diet reduces these negative symptoms and improves the child's ability to cope.

A recent study[1] by researchers at Penn State documented survey data gathered from parents of autistic children regarding the effectiveness of a gluten-free, casein-free diet on children diagnosed with autism. The survey results suggested that parents who completely eliminated both gluten and casein from their child's diet reported the most benefit.

The good news is that you and our health care provider can eliminate these other problems once you conclude the symptoms are caused by gluten intolerance. You can begin to change your diet and experience a great deal of improvement in all of these symptoms.

If you have symptoms of gluten intolerance it's important to speak with a health care provider to rule out other health problems with similar symptoms. If you have an autistic child, don't postpone getting a specialist involved. And once you've narrowed the source of problems down to gluten intolerance, you have the power to improve your lifestyle and health rapidly.

-------------------

# Gluten Sensitivity vs. Celiac Disease vs. Crohn's Disease vs. Irritable Bowel Syndrome

There's a lot of talk today about gluten intolerance or allergies and having problems digesting it. But what's the difference between having a little sensitivity to gluten and having a health condition that requires medical attention? Let's take a look at some of the different conditions you've heard of.

**Celiac disease** is a serious disease that comes from an autoimmune response to gluten in the body. People who have celiac disease need to eat a gluten-free diet. Basically, gluten intolerance and celiac disease are one in the same with varying degrees of problematic symptoms. The symptoms of celiac disease range from diarrhea, constipation and gas to anemia, irritability, or frequent nose bleeds.

When you have celiac disease, the lining of your small intestine actually becomes damaged. This is the part of your digestive system that absorbs nutrients from your food. Continued problems with celiac can actually cause you to become malnourished.

Malnourishment from celiac can further cause symptoms such as fatigue, problems with appetite, and even nausea and vomiting. No one knows exactly why this happens, but we do know that following a gluten-free diet will control it.

**Crohn's disease** is another painful condition that takes place in the intestinal tract. This is an autoimmune disease that causes symptoms similar to celiac disease, but it's not related to gluten. However, eating gluten-free likely will help the Crohn's sufferer as well. A diagnosis of Crohn's will come by ruling out other conditions.

If you have Crohn's, you may want to avoid foods that cause problems with gas and bloating for you – they can be different for different people. However, gluten isn't thought to be the culprit, but may be impacting this condition. Crohn's is treated by improving diet, taking medications, and even surgery.

**Irritable Bowel Syndrome (IBS)** is another disorder of the digestive tract. It has a wide range of symptoms such as diarrhea and constipation. Some people with irritable bowel syndrome have problems with frequent and urgent bowel movements. While others will suffer from chronic constipation.

There's no one cause for IBS, rather it's a collection of symptoms that aren't caused by any specific thing. Your diet will need to change based on what's best for you, but gluten isn't the sole culprit for this problem. Eating gluten-free may help though.

With **gluten sensitivity**, you may experience mild problems such as bloating and gas when you eat foods that contain gluten. However, you're not likely to have a violent response or malnourishment as people with celiac disease experience.

Whether you have gluten sensitivity or celiac disease, it makes sense to eat a gluten-free diet so you can eliminate all of your symptoms. It can be uncomfortable and embarrassing to have problems with your digestive system. In the case of celiac, eliminating gluten can literally save your life.

There are other health conditions that might also benefit from a gluten-free diet. One of the greatest benefits of eating a gluten-free diet can be weight loss as previously mentioned. This weight loss is likely to be modest. When you go on a gluten-free diet you are often removing high calorie foods and snacks. Because gluten is known to cause inflammation in many people, if you have certain health conditions, this inflammation will exacerbate your symptoms. Some conditions that can benefit from a gluten free diet are multiple sclerosis, chronic fatigue syndrome, and other auto-immune diseases.

Diabetes is another condition that can often be helped by eating a gluten-free diet. Foods that are high in gluten are also often high in simple carbohydrates. These foods tend to cause insulin and blood sugar levels to go haywire.

Infertility, especially if it's caused by polycystic ovarian syndrome, can be alleviated by letting go of gluten. Women who have insulin resistance and foods that are high in gluten tend to cause problems with blood sugar leading to hormonal imbalance.

Many cancers can also be prevented it is believed by eating a healthy diet that's high in organic vegetables, and modest fruit and low in foods that contain high amounts of gluten. That's because most foods that contain large amounts of gluten are also high in sugar (which cancer cells love), saturated fats, and additives.

A gluten-free diet can also lead to lower levels of cholesterol and decrease your risk of heart disease and stroke. You'll be eliminating many unhealthy foods and focusing on adding healthful foods such as lean proteins, fruits, and vegetables. As Hippocrates so wisely stated thousands of years ago, "let food be thy medicine and medicine be thy food".

## What is it About Gluten that Makes You Ill?

If you have celiac disease or gluten intolerance, you may wonder what it is about gluten that makes you sick. In modern times more and more people are affected by problems with gluten and have turned to a gluten-free diet in order to regain wellness.

Gluten is a protein that's found in grains such as wheat, rye, and barley. This protein is abundant in foods that contain these grains. And while it seems pretty innocuous it can cause some major problems in the body. In recent studies gluten has been shown to increase zonulin, a protein that increases intestinal permeability of the tight junctions between cell walls of the digestive tract. This was discovered by Dr. Alessio Fasano at the University of Maryland School of Medicine in 2000. Gliadin is the glycoprotein in gluten containing grains that is responsible for activating zonulin.

Just like with any allergy, someone who has an allergy to gluten can have a serious response. The body sees the protein as a foreign invader that needs to be destroyed and removed from the body. When you have an allergy to pollen, it causes you to sneeze, have watery eyes, and can lead to problems with your sinuses. That's your body's response to ridding your body of it. With a gluten allergy, your digestive system is doing the same type of thing – trying to attack it and get rid of it.

Your body's immune system is very complex and very advanced. It produced antibodies that are designed to specifically fight foreign invaders. When you have a gluten allergy, your body produces antibodies that are marked to fight the protein.

When the gluten enters your body, it's immediately recognized by the antibodies and your immune system is alerted that it's time to make a full-scale attack. For some people this results in some diarrhea or even constipation.

For others, the allergy is much more severe and actually causes damage to the lining of the small intestine. This form of the allergy is known as celiac disease. The good news is that while there's no cure for this illness, it can be controlled through diet.

By eating a gluten-free diet, you deprive your body of the allergen. If you don't expose it to gluten you won't experience symptoms. And fortunately, it's easier to establish and maintain a "gluten free" diet today than in years past.

There are many products on the market that will even allow you to enjoy foods that are usually made from wheat, barley, or rye. As you eliminate the gluten from your body, you'll begin to feel better and better.

No one knows for sure what causes the sensitivity to gluten, though it may be genetic. Other culprits believed to be contributing to gluten sensitivity are the introduction of genetically modified foods and the overuse of pesticides and herbicides. In the end, if you have problems processing gluten it's best to stay away from it. Gluten can cause serious and devastating symptoms if you ignore it.

# DIY Testing for Gluten Sensitivity

People concerned about gluten proteins causing problems can perform some basic DIY testing for gluten sensitivity which will help you get closer to the specific cause of health problems and allow them to move toward permanent relief.

So is there a way to perform a do-it-yourself test for gluten sensitivity? While the preferred option is to have testing performed by a doctor or a specialist in allergies and immunology, you may not want to spend the time or money getting that done until you've ruled out other possible conditions.

One thing you can do is keep a food diary that includes symptoms. You can track exactly what you're eating and write down any experiences you have with bloating, gas, constipation, or diarrhea. You should also note symptoms such as fatigue and headaches.

Over time, you'll begin to see patterns developing if you have sensitivity to gluten. For example, you may notice that every time you eat bread you have bloating. You may also want to try a gluten-free bread alternative to see how your body reacts. Keeping a daily food journal will prove very useful should you end up going to an allergist or specialist.

The pulse test can actually help you determine if you have an allergy to gluten or to any food. You'll want to log your resting pulse rate at several times throughout the day and record it. Then you'll want to record your pulse after eating different, specific foods.

The idea is that when you eat foods for which you have an allergy or sensitivity, your pulse will actually speed up as your immune response kicks in. You'll want to do this over a long period of time. It's also important to remember that movement, stress, and other factors can cause similar changes.

Eliminating gluten can also help you to decide if you're intolerant to it. If you avoid gluten for a time and notice that you're feeling much better, you're probably someone who has a gluten sensitivity.

If restricting your diet from gluten products doesn't give you much relief from symptoms, there may be multiple food intolerances or other diseases involved. Therefore, it's important to make an appointment with your health care provider. He or she can verify the allergy or sensitivity through more sophisticated testing. It is important to understand that many health care providers are unaware or knowledgeable of some of the tests that are available today to check for a sensitivity to gluten or other foods. One thing to be aware of is when you eliminate gluten from your diet with your DIY gluten testing, you'll make it difficult for professional medical tests to pick up your celiac disease. If you're going to meet with your health care provider, it's best to revert to your old eating habits to achieve more relevant results from your tests. Better yet, if you have already gone gluten-free and feel better, you have your answer. Since many conventionally trained health care providers are unfamiliar with ways to test for gluten sensitivity, you might want to seek out a provider trained in natural or functional medicine. Most are familiar with ways to look for gluten sensitivity. Most cases of celiac disease can be diagnosed by a gastroenterologist or specialist of the digestive tract.

# What is a Gluten-Free Diet?

In order to get an understanding of what a gluten-free diet is all about, it helps to first know what gluten is. Gluten is a protein that's found in grains such as wheat, barley, and rye.

Some people have an allergy to this protein and eating foods with gluten cause symptoms such as diarrhea, constipation, vomiting, and gas. As you can imagine, it's important to eliminate gluten if you have such an allergy.

Living with a gluten-free diet was once a difficult feat, but these days it's pretty easy to find gluten-free recipes and products. If you wish to eliminate gluten from your diet, it helps to evaluate what you're eating now.

Items made with whole wheat or white flour all contain gluten. This means most cookies, cakes, breads, muffins, pastas, and cereals contain it. It is also hidden in many processed foods. To eat gluten-free, you'll need to replace those items with gluten-free versions or eliminate grains from your diet.

Some grains are safe to eat. Oats, for example, don't naturally contain gluten. However, it's important to look for oats labeled as "gluten-free" because they can become exposed to other grains when they're processed.

There are many gluten free flours now on the market that you can use in backing. These include brown rice, millet, buckwheat, sweet white rice, corn, and almond flours. Almond flour is also lower in carbohydrates. You can make your own flour blends or purchase one of the ready-made all purpose flour blends as well. There are several to choose from.

Many people diagnosed with gluten sensitivity or celiac disease fear that they won't be able to enjoy the foods they love. But a quick trip to Whole Foods or even the local supermarket can open up the possibilities for a variety of food options. A health food store is another option for gluten-free products. However, if you can access the internet, by all means check out the gluten-free items on Amazon.com. Gluten-free does not necessarily mean healthy, so choose wisely.

If you haven't used Amazon before it is the Mega of Megastore with everything from tropical fish food to diatomaceous earth products. It offers great selections of gluten-free products and often your order is shipped FREE. Amazon is truly the answer to stress-free shopping for special dietary needs.

Mixes for gluten-free brownies, cookies, muffins, and breads are readily available but not necessarily healthy. Healthy naturally gluten-free alternatives include nuts, eggs, vegetables, and fruit. You'll need to check the labels of everything you eat when you're beginning a gluten-free diet. This little protein can turn up in unexpected places. For example, it can be found in soups, salad dressings, frozen meals, and other ready-to-eat foods.

It's important to look at the ingredients to see if wheat, rye, and/or barley are on the label. Many products will advertise that they're gluten-free to make it easier for you to get your shopping done. You can still eat many foods you enjoy when you go gluten-free.

Anything that doesn't contain gluten and hasn't been exposed to it is safe to eat. Rice, fruits, vegetables, most dairy products, and meats are safe to enjoy. While it may be difficult to eliminate gluten at first, it becomes easier as you continue to practice a gluten-free lifestyle. Eliminating your symptoms is great motivation for determining what path to follow for a gluten-free diet.

## There is a great site at

http://glutenfreegirl.com/2012/07/how-to-make-a-gluten-free-all-purpose-flour-mix/

where a woman shares her tips in a live audio file. Simply press the 'go' arrow and there she is explaining what she does to make her own gluten-free flour. In the video, she explains her recipe using sorghum, millet and sweet rice flours, along with potato starch. Are you beginning to see a pattern here? All the recipes contain flour and starch, as the whole grain flour is chockfull of protein, the added starch to the blend is what holds it all together, plus it adds a 'white' component to the mix, appearing more like most gluten-based flour, so your recipes, too, will come out looking like you used 'regular' flour. Again, this site is geared to those who want to experiment with their own gluten-free flour blends.

The site goes on to list by categories whole grain flours, white flour starches, nut flours, and bean flours. Each category has at least four options so for anyone feeling experimental can surely come up with a gluten-free flour made from a variety of sources. Eventually you may hit on a blend that suits your tastes and the one you can call your own.

## 4 Tips For Beginners of Gluten-Free Cooking

**First**, experiment, experiment and experiment. There is a learning curve when you first start with Gluten-free cooking, but once you get some practice and experience you will become an expert about what works and what does not.

**Second**, stay with it and don't get discouraged. There will be failed recipes because you have to learn which flour combinations work best, but it just takes practice and testing. It's best to get guidance from recipe books or online guides when first starting out so you don't waste time re-inventing the wheel.

**Third**, begin with simple recipes and learn the basics. As you get more experienced and master those, you can move onto the more complicated dishes.

**Fourth**, when you pinpoint the perfect flour combinations to match your taste, stick with it and likely it will work for all your cooking and baking needs.

## Fad or Health Movement

One can certainly understand why moving to a diet free of gluten can help relieve serious health conditions caused by an allergic reaction to gluten. There is a growing trend for people who don't suffer from gluten intolerance or celiac disease to abstain from gluten products even though they don't experience distress after consuming gluten products. The bottom line is the gluten protein is very hard to digest and is rough on your gut. When your stomach is not functioning well, your entire body will not feel as healthy as it should because it simply cannot absorb all of the proper nutrients from the foods you eat. The result is a body that is not nourished efficiently, and one that is more susceptible to illnesses.

# Advantages of a Gluten-Free Diet

For some people, gluten sensitivity makes eating gluten-free a necessity. But even if you don't have a sensitivity, a gluten-free diet can be beneficial. One of the greatest benefits of eating gluten-free is to remove an overload of carbohydrates from your diet. Consuming fewer carbs can help people lose weight. Many of the high sugar carbohydrates that lead to weight gain also contain gluten. So if you remove gluten from your diet, you'll also reduce your caloric intake.

A gluten-free diet is naturally more dependent on fruits, vegetables, and proteins to get your nutrition. You'll be avoiding many products that are processed such as breads, cereals, cookies, and cakes that can lead to weight gain.

You'll also improve your health. When you eat more fruits and vegetables, you'll increase the fiber in your diet. This can help you to lower your cholesterol, regulate your digestive system, and lower your risk of developing diabetes.

A gluten-free diet can also help you to reduce your risk of developing some cancers. A diet high in fiber, low in fat and chemicals from processing and high in vitamins can help your body fight off cancer.

Your immune system will also function better when you have a diet that's high in antioxidants that come from fruits and vegetables. You'll have fewer problems with colds, flu, and other infections.

If weight loss and improved health aren't enough to convince you, you might also consider that a gluten-free diet can help you to have increased energy. Many people who find that they feel sluggish or run down find that those feelings go away as they remove gluten from their diet.

Grains that are high in starch often lead to inflammations within the body. The more the refined the grain is, the more potential there is for inflammation. Unbleached white flour is much more inflammatory than even processed wheat flour. On the other hand, gluten free foods such as fresh vegetables and healthy types of fat can actually help to reduce inflammation. Patients who suffer with arthritis, asthma, cardiovascular disease, and even allergies have all shown improvement while on a gluten free diet.

Some health conditions have also shown improvement by eliminating gluten from the diet as noted earlier. For example, Hashimoto's, multiple sclerosis, autism, and irritable bowel syndrome have all shown improvement in people when they switch to a gluten-free diet.

Some people have sensitivities to gluten even if they don't have celiac disease or an outright allergy. You may feel bloated, gassy, or have problems with diarrhea and constipation if you eat gluten. By eliminating gluten you can be free of these problems.

Athletes who depend on a diet that affords a high nutritional value often opt for a gluten-free diet simply because gluten inhibits the body's ability to absorb minerals. Gluten grains are not properly digested making it very difficult for the body to gain any nutrition from these foods. While you may believe you are eating a diet rich in key nutrients, iron, and calcium, gluten grains that are eaten will actually block your body's ability to absorb everything you need.

Here's a reason to frown. Gluten contains a phosphorus mineral called phytate. Phytate acids are linked to an increase in tooth decay because they block other minerals from being absorbed which then cause bacteria to feed on starches in your mouth. This leads to gingivitis and tooth decay.

Do you suffer from oily skin or frustrated with acne? Try removing gluten from your diet. Gluten is a carbohydrate and carbs are broken down into sugars during the digestion process. When you have sugars in your bloodstream your pancreas generates more insulin which in turn causes other hormones to fire. Ultimately all this increases the amount of oil produced by the oil glands in your skin and that leads to more acne. If you were blaming the fatty cheese on your pizza for causing a breakout of acne, the culprit may have been the pizza dough.

If you're considering whether or not to eliminate gluten from your diet, you should consider that it has many benefits. You can gradually begin to eliminate products that contain gluten – it doesn't have to be done all at once, though is encouraged to get the most benefit.

# Five Steps to Transition into a Gluten-Free Lifestyle

At first, the thought of adopting a diet free of gluten can be overwhelming, but it can be easy if you follow these 5 steps to transition into a gluten-free lifestyle. Unless you have celiac disease which may require you to move rapidly or even cold turkey on gluten, you can slowly move toward a gluten-free life if you are overwhelmed at the prospect of going "cold turkey".

**#1 Get the Family Involved**

Moms and dads who are the breadwinners and bread makers, but who are also the gluten intolerant will need help from their spouses and kids. You don't have to force everyone into the same diet plan, but it will make food preparation much easier. As you start to transition gluten-free recipes and products into the daily menu, look for positive feedback from the family. If you hit a winner, stick with it.

### #2 Zero in on Gluten-Based Products

Gluten is a protein found in wheat, rye, and barley. So it will obviously be found in breads and other foods made of those grains. However, it also pops up in unexpected places.

It's important to check labels and look for gluten. You'll be surprised what products include gluten as a base. Many soups, sauces, and gravies include gluten even though you might not expect to find them there.

Don't overlook the dressing you pour on salads. They are notorious for having gluten as a base thickener. The only way to know is to check the label. Check your pantry and make sure to check labels when you shop.

### #3 Start Eliminating Gluten Foods

Put on your research hat and find out where to buy gluten-free products. Consider eliminating one gluten product at a time. Instead of throwing out everything containing gluten, try choosing one product that you can live without. For example, you might want to get rid of your current cereal and look for one that's gluten-free.

After you've had time to get used to your new cereal, you can eliminate another product. Trying to do it all at once may be too overwhelming and can also shock your taste buds. But if you focus on one food at a time, you'll have a smoother transition. Just know that you will not likely completely resolve your symptoms until all gluten is out of your diet.

**#4 Focus On Adding Gluten-Free Food Items You Enjoy**

Instead of thinking about all the things you "can't" have, pay attention to the things you can have. Especially make room for treats in your diet that are gluten-free, but you really love. It's all too common to focus on what you're eliminating rather than understanding that there are many tasty foods that don't contain gluten.

Look for recipes that are gluten-free and have fun trying new things. Start a local gluten-free group and exchange recipes. Facebook is a great way to connect with others who are going gluten-free.

### #5 Identify Resources Offering Gluten-Free Products

Look for gluten-free alternatives to your favorite menu items. You'll notice that non-gluten products have a different texture, but over time you'll grow to enjoy them especially since you can have a sandwich, pizza or pasta and not suffer from gassy bloat afterwards.

Don't forget to shop at Amazon for alternatives. You'll find loads of gluten-free. When ordering from Amazon it really pays to order the bulk items. In fact, chances are you'll notice that the price per unit is cheaper than the single unit items of the same product sold in a natural food or grocery store. The bottom line is you're you are going to pay more for non-gluten products, but on Amazon you only need an order of $25 and shipping is free. That's gas you don't have to burn chasing around town for gluten groceries.

You don't need to break the bank and try every item at once. Think about substituting one thing at a time. For example, give the pasta a try but wait to try gluten-free bread until you've gotten used to the pasta.

Finally, pay attention to how eliminating gluten makes you feel. When you begin to feel frustrated with making the switch to a gluten-free diet it can help to pay attention to your improved health and energy.

Giving up gluten doesn't have to be a painful experience. If you take your time and focus on why you're doing it, you can enjoy the process. Following these five steps to transition into a gluten-free diet can help you to be successful.

# Gluten-Free Grains

If you're looking to eliminate gluten from your diet, you need to know which gluten free grains are safe to add to your diet. While gluten is found in many foods, there are many that are free of the gluten protein. It helps to know where to turn to when you're eliminating gluten.

First, it's important to know where gluten is found. In general, you'll find it in foods made from wheat, barley, and rye. Gluten is a protein that's found in these grains and is responsible for the way dough stretches.

But there are several grains that don't include gluten as mentioned earlier. These grains will make it possible for you to enjoy grains without dealing with the adverse side effects that can sometimes come along with gluten. Let's look at some of these gluten-free grains closer.

**Rice** is a gluten-free grain. You can cook and eat rice as a side dish, but it can also be part of many gluten-free products. For example, there are cereals and noodles made from rice that are gluten-free.

**Oats** can also be eaten as part of a gluten-free diet. Be careful and check that the oats you eat aren't contaminated with other grains. Look for oats that bear "gluten-free" on the label. There are breads, pancake mixes, and oat flours that are gluten-free.

**Corn** is found in many products and is also gluten-free. You may see the term "corn gluten" on a label but that isn't the same as the gluten found in wheat, barley, and rye. You can enjoy many foods that contain corn and still keep gluten at bay.

**Quinoa** is a grain that's gained popularity in recent times. This grain can be found in many products and can be used in side dishes, salads, and casseroles. It's also touted to have other health properties that make it an excellent addition to your diet.

**Buckwheat** is another grain you can enjoy when you're living gluten-free. Despite its name, it isn't really wheat and it doesn't contain gluten. It's common in many Asian dishes and it can be a main ingredient in gluten free noodles.

Another grain that's commonly used in Asian countries is **millet**. It can be found in porridges and even alcoholic beverages can be made from it. Millet flour can also be used to make flatbreads.

You may have heard of **sorghum** before. This is a grain that's primarily used for making molasses but it can also be found in some alcohols. It's another product that's gluten free and safe for you to eat. White sorghum is also being milled into flour now as well.

Eating a gluten-free diet doesn't mean you have to avoid all grains, though limiting grains is overall good for your health. There are many gluten free grains that can help you to have a healthy and satisfying diet without having to suffer from digestive problems or weight gain.

# Avoid These Foods and Products

When you're working on living with a gluten-free diet, you'll want to avoid these foods and products that can have detrimental health effects for you. Some of these products are obvious, but others might not be obvious to you.

First, it's always important to avoid the grains that contain gluten. This includes wheat, barley, and rye and any products made from them. You're most likely to find these gluten grains in cereals, breads, cookies, and cakes made from these grains. I know you have read this before but it is important to understand which grains contain gluten.

You'll want to be careful when eating any pastas or crackers that might contain gluten – most of them do. Unless this type of food is labeled as "gluten free" you'll just want to assume it contains it.

It's also important to avoid drinking beer. If you don't know much about its processing this might seem odd, but it's actually made from barley which contains gluten. Other alcoholic beverages such as wine, whiskey, and other liqueurs are generally okay. Just check the label.

Canned and processed foods such as soups, gravies, and sauces should also be carefully scrutinized. Many of them contain wheat gluten even if they don't seem to be something that would have grain in them.

Items such as salad dressings, ketchup, and lunch meats can often be found to have gluten in them. You might also find it in instant drinks such as coffee and hot chocolate and in your favorite candy. Always check the labels before you eat something.

Wheat flour is often used as a thickener for products so make sure to check the label before purchasing any kind of processed food. More of them contain gluten than you might expect and you don't want to inadvertently ingest gluten.

Check your medicine cabinet to make sure you're gluten-free there as well. Many capsules, tablets, and gel caps are made from sources that contain gluten. You might be accidentally encountering gluten while you're trying to improve your health.

Celiac disease and gluten intolerance often go hand in hand with lactose intolerance. If you're someone who has been diagnosed with celiac, you should talk with your health care provider about eliminating dairy products as well.

Once your symptoms have subsided and you've eliminated gluten, you might be able to reintroduce milk products. It is often best to avoid dairy permanently, just like the gluten.

Oats are okay to have if they're not contaminated with wheat products. However, many oats are processed in factories that also process gluten containing grains. Make sure that you purchase only oats that are labeled as "gluten free".

# Handy Gluten Free Grocery List Visual

You can download this handy gluten-free visual called the "Gluten Free Grocery List" and then print out a couple of copies to keep with you when you go shopping or post it in the kitchen. You'll quickly learn what foods to avoid with this handy graphic.

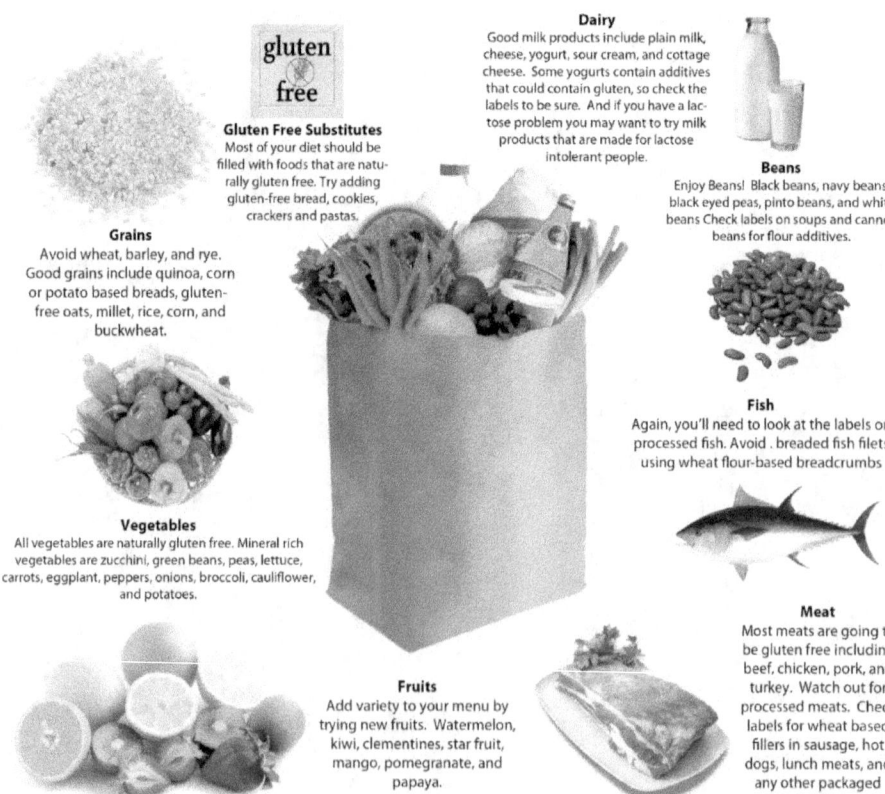

**Gluten Free Substitutes**
Most of your diet should be filled with foods that are naturally gluten free. Try adding gluten-free bread, cookies, crackers and pastas.

**Grains**
Avoid wheat, barley, and rye. Good grains include quinoa, corn or potato based breads, gluten-free oats, millet, rice, corn, and buckwheat.

**Dairy**
Good milk products include plain milk, cheese, yogurt, sour cream, and cottage cheese. Some yogurts contain additives that could contain gluten, so check the labels to be sure. And if you have a lactose problem you may want to try milk products that are made for lactose intolerant people.

**Beans**
Enjoy Beans! Black beans, navy beans, black eyed peas, pinto beans, and white beans Check labels on soups and canned beans for flour additives.

**Fish**
Again, you'll need to look at the labels on processed fish. Avoid . breaded fish filets using wheat flour-based breadcrumbs

**Vegetables**
All vegetables are naturally gluten free. Mineral rich vegetables are zucchini, green beans, peas, lettuce, carrots, eggplant, peppers, onions, broccoli, cauliflower, and potatoes.

**Fruits**
Add variety to your menu by trying new fruits. Watermelon, kiwi, clementines, star fruit, mango, pomegranate, and papaya.

**Meat**
Most meats are going to be gluten free including beef, chicken, pork, and turkey. Watch out for processed meats. Check labels for wheat based fillers in sausage, hot dogs, lunch meats, and any other packaged meats.

# Conclusion

The best way to manage gluten intolerance is with a gluten-free diet. Going gluten free means removing grains like wheat, rye, barley, and triticale which contain the protein gluten. These grains are found in different formats such as flour, thickeners and bases. Gluten based products are used as an additive in many food products.

Once gluten is removed from the diet, your digestive system begins to heal allowing it to perform as a high performance system instead of one that is constantly fighting against the negative effects of gluten. Gluten proteins inhibit the absorption of vital nutrients.

Your stomach is an important part of the digestive system, but once food passes through the gut the intestines are in charge. Your intestines are responsible for absorbing the minerals and vitamins from digested food. Once you remove gluten from your diet, the intestines can better handle normal absorption of nutrients. This is essential for the body to obtain all the vital nutrients it needs to sustain itself.

You'll find the change to a gluten-free diet will not only make you feel a lot healthier, but you will enjoy higher levels of energy, be able to concentrate and focus better and look forward to each day free of the symptoms associated with gluten intolerance.

# Gluten-Free Food Lists

Enjoy all fresh fruits, vegetables, nuts, fish, shellfish, and meats as long as they are not processed (i.e., mixes, sauces, canned, meals). Evaluate ingredient labels whenever you try out a new a processed food.

Oats are gluten-free, but may be grown or processed with wheat during. This contamination leaves oats as a questionable item. Look for oat products that are gluten-free.

Don't forget to download your gluten free shopping guide. If you are wondering which restaurants offer gluten-free selections, just click on this link to see if your favorite restaurant is on the list. If your restaurant is not on the list, don't despair as many restaurants are adding gluten-free dishes every day. Just call and ask them.

The lists below are not all inclusive, but include popular food items and common food additives. When in doubt, put it back on the shelf and do your own due diligence.

# Gluten-Free Fruits & Vegetables

**Fruits**

Apple
Apricot
Avocado
Banana
Bilberry
Blackberry
Blackcurrant
Blueberry
Breadfruit
Cantaloupe
Cherimoya
Cherry
Clementine
Currant
Damson
Date
Dragonfruit
Durian
Eggplant
Elderberry
Feijoa
Gooseberry
Grape
Grapefruit
Guava
Honeydew melon
Huckleberry
Jackfruit
Jambul
Kiwi fruit
Kumquat
Legume

Mandarine
Mango
Melon
Nectarine
Orange
Peach
Pear
Physalis
Pineapple
Pitaya
Plum/prune (dried plum)
Pomegranate
Pomelo
Purple Mangosteen
Raisin
Rambutan
Raspberry
Redcurrant
Rock melon
Salal berry
Satsuma
Star fruit
Strawberry
Tangerine
Tomato
Ugli fruit
Watermelon
Watermelon--see melon
Western raspberry (blackcap)
Williams pear or Bartlett pear
Ziziphus mauritiana

Lemon
Lime
Lychee

# Gluten-Free Grains, Dairy, Meats, Fish, Shellfish & Nuts

## Grains
Amaranth
Buckwheat
Corn
Millet
Montina (Indian rice grass)
Oats** opt for a Gluten-Free product
Quinoa
Rice
Sorghum
Teff
Wild Rice

## Dairy (always check labels)
Check for lactose intolerance
Plain milk, but avoid flavored milk
Plain yogurt is usually safe, check flavored yogurts
Eggs
Butter
Cottage Cheese
Ice Cream and Sherberts proceed with caution

Non-processed cheese, but watch out for "beer washed" cheeses

**Meats, Fish, Shellfish, Nuts**

All non-processed, otherwise check additive list and ingredients

# Gluten-Free Vegetables

## Vegetables

| | |
|---|---|
| Artichoke | Melons |
| Asparagus | Mushrooms |
| Aubergene | Okra |
| Beans | Onions |
| Beet | Pak Choi |
| Broccoli | Parsnips |
| Brussels sprouts | Peas |
| Cabbage | Peppers |
| Carrot | Potatoes |
| Cauliflower | Pumpkins |
| Celeriac | Radicchio |
| Celery | Radish |
| Chard | Rhubarb |
| Chicory | Rutabaga |
| Collards | Shallots |
| Corn | Spinach |
| Cress | Squash |
| Cucumbers | Swede |
| Gourds | Sweetcorn |
| Jerusalem Artichoke | Sweet potato |
| | Tomatoes (fruit, vegetable, |
| Kales | whatever) |
| Kohlrabi | Turnips |
| Leek | Watercress |
| Lettuce | Watermelon |
| | Yams |

# Gluten-Free Food Additives

## A

Acacia Gum
Acacia Gum
Acesulfame K
Acesulfame Potassium
Acetanisole
Acetophenone
Acorn Quercus
Adipic Acid
Adzuki Bean
Agar
Agave
Albumen
Alfalfa
Algae
Algin
Alginate
Alginic Acid
Alkalized Cocoa
Allicin
Almond Nut
Alpha-amylase
Alpha-lactalbumin
Aluminum
Amaranth
Ambergris

Ammonium Hydroxide
Ammonium Phosphate
Ammonium Sulphate
Amylopectin
Amylose
Annatto
Annatto Color
Apple Cider Vinegar
Arabic Gum
Arrowroot
Artichokes
Artificial Butter Flavor
Ascorbic Acid
Aspartame (IBS symptoms)
Aspartic Acid
Aspic
Astragalus Gummifer
Autolyzed Yeast Extract
Avena Sativia (Oats3)
Avidin
Azodicarbonamide

## Gluten-Free Food Additives

# B

Baking Soda
Balsamic Vinegar
Bean Romano (Chickpea)
Bean Tepary
Bean, Adzuki
Bean, Hyacinth
Bean, Lentil
Bean, Mung
Beans

Beeswax
Benzoic acid
Besan (Chickpea)
Beta Carotene
Beta Glucan (from Oats)
Betaine
BHA
BHT
Bicarbonate of Soda
Biotin
Blue Cheese
Brown Sugar
Buckwheat
Butter (check additives)
Butyl Compounds
Butylated Hydroxyanisole

## Gluten-Free Food Additives
# C
Calcium Acetate
Calcium Carbonate
Calcium Caseinate
Calcium Chloride
Calcium Disodium
Calcium Hydroxide
Calcium Lactate
Calcium Pantothenate
Calcium Phosphate
Calcium Propionate
Calcium Silicate
Calcium Sorbate
Calcium Stearate
Caclium Stearoyl Lactylate
Calcium Sulfate
Camphor
Cane sugar
Cane Vinegar

Canola (Rapeseed)
Canola Oil (Rapeseed Oil)
Caprylic Acid
Carageenan Chondrus Crispus
Carbonated Water
Carboxymethyl Cellulose
Carmine
Carnauba Wax
Carob Bean
Carob Bean Gum
Carob Flour
Carrageenan
Casein
Cassava Manihot Esculenta
Castor Oil
Catalase
Cellulose Ether
Chestnuts
Chickpea (Channa)
Chlorella
Chocolate Liquor
Choline Chloride
Chromium Citrate
Chymosin
Citric Acid
Citrus Red No. 2
Cochineal
Cocoa
Cocoa Butter
Coconut
Coconut Vinegar
Collagen
Colloidal Silicon Dioxide
Confectioner's Glaze
Copernicia Cerifera
Copper Sulphate

Corn
Corn Flour
Corn Gluten
Corn Masa Flour
Corn Meal
Corn Flour
Corn Starch
Corn Sugar
Corn Sugar Vinegar
Corn Syrup
Corn Syrup Solids
Corn Swetener
Corn Vinegar
Corn Zein
Cortisone
Cotton Seed
Cotton Seed Oil
Cowitch
Cowpea
Cream of Tartar
Crospovidone
Curds
Cyanocobalamin
Cysteine, L

## Gluten-Free Food Additives
# D
Dal (Lentils)
D-Alpha-tocopherol
Dasheen Flour (Taro)
Dates
D-Calcium Pantothenate

Delactosed Whey
Demineralized Whey
Desamidocollagen
Dextran

Dextrose
Diglycerides
Dioctyl Sodium
Dioctyl Sodium Solfosuccinate
Dipotassium Phosphate
Disodium Guanylate
Disodium Inosinate
Disodium Phosphate
Distilled Alcohols
Distilled Vinegar
Distilled White Vinegar
Dutch Processed Cocoa

## Gluten-Free Food Additives

## E

EDTA (Ethylenediaminetetraacetic Acid)
Eggs
Egg Yolks
Elastin
Ester Gum
Ethyl Alcohol
Ethylenediaminetetraacetic Acid
Ethyl Maltol
Ethyl Vanillin
Expeller Pressed Canola Oil

## F

FD&C Blue No. 1 Dye
FD&C Blue No. 1 Lake
FD&C Blue No. 2 Dye
FD&C Blue No. 2 Lake
FD&C Green No. 3 Dye
FD&C Green No. 3 Lake
FD&C Red No. 3 Dye
FD&C Red No. 40 Dye
FD&C Red No. 40 Lake
FD&C Yellow No. 5 Dye

FD&C Yellow No. 6 Dye

FD&C Yellow No. 6 Lake
Ferric Orthophosphate
Ferrous Gluconate
Ferrous Fumerate
Ferrous Lactate
Ferrous Sulfate
Fish (fresh)
Flaked Rice
Flax
Folacin
Folate
Folic Acid-Folacin
Formaldehyde
Fructose
Fruit Vinegar
Fumaric Acid

## Gluten-Free Food Additives
## G
Galactose
Garbanzo Beans
Gelatin
Glucoamylase
Gluconolactone
Glucose
Glucose Syrup
Glutamate (free)
Glutamic Acid
Glutamine (amino acid)
Glutinous Rice
Glutinous Rice Flour
Glycerides
Glycerin
Glycerol Monooleate
Glycol Monosterate
Glycol
Glycolic acid

Gram flour (chick peas)

Grape Skin Extract
Grits, Corn
Guar Gum
Gum Acacia
Gum Arabic
Gum Base
Gum Tragacanth

## Gluten-Free Food Additives
# H
Hemp
Hemp Seeds
Herbs
Herb Vinegar
Hexanedioic Acid
High Fructose Corn Syrup
Hominy
Honey
Hops
Horseradish (Pure)
Hyacinth Bean
Hydrogen Peroxide
Hydrolyzed Caseinate
Hydrolyzed Meat Protein
Hydrolyzed Soy Protein
Hydroxypropyl Cellulose
Hydroxypropyl Methylcellulose
Hypromellose

## Gluten-Free Food Additives
# I
Illepe
Iodine
Inulin
Invert Sugar
Iron Ammonium Citrate

Isinglass
Isolated Soy Protein
Isomalt

## Gluten-Free Food Additives

# J
Job's Tears
Jowar (Sorghum)

# K
Karaya Gum
Kasha (roasted buckwheat)
Keratin
K-Carmine Color
K-Gelatin
Koshihikari (rice)
Kudzu
Kudzu Root Starch

## Gluten-Free Food Additives

# L
Lactalbumin Phosphate
Lactase
Lactic Acid
Lactitol
Lactose
Lactulose
Lanolin
Lard
L-cysteine
Lecithin
Lemon Grass
Lentils
Licorice
Licorice Extract
Lipase
L-leucine

L-lysine
L-methionine
Locust Bean Gum
L-tryptophan

## Gluten-Free Food Additives

# M

Magnesium Carbonate
Magnesium Hydroxide
Magnesium Oxide
Maize
Maize Waxy
Malic Acid
Maltitol
Maltodextrin
Maltol
Manganese Sulfate
Manioc
Masa
Masa Flour
Masa Harina
Meat (fresh)
Medium Chain Triglycerides
Menhaden Oil
Methyl Cellulose2
Microcrystalline Cellulose
Micro-particulated Egg White Protein
Milk
Milk Protein Isolate
Millet
Milo (Sorghum)
Mineral Oil
Mineral Salts
Molybdenum Amino Acid Chelate
Monocalcium Phosphate
Monoglycerides
Mono and Diglycerides
Monopotassium Phosphate
monosaccharides

Monosodium Glutamate (MSG)

Monostearates
MSG
Mung Bean
Musk
Mustard Flour
Myristic Acid

## Gluten-Free Food Additives
# N
Natural Smoke Flavor
Niacin-Niacinamide
Neotame
Niacin
Niacinamide
Nitrates
Nitrous Oxide
Non-fat Milk
Nut, Acron
Nut, Almond

# O
Oats3
Oils and Fats
Oleic Acid
Oleoresin
Olestra
Oleyl Alcohol/Oil
Orange B
Oryzanol

## Gluten-Free Food Additives
# P
Palmitic Acid
Pantothenic Acid
Papain
Paprika

Paraffin

## Gluten-Free Food Additives

Peas
Pea - Chick
Pea - Cow
Pea Flour
Pea Starch
Peanuts
Peanut Flour
Pectin
Pectinase
Peppermint Oil
Peppers
Pepsin
Peru Balsam
Petrolatum
PGPR (Polyglycerol Polyricinoleate)
Phenylalanine
Phosphoric Acid
Phosphoric Glycol
Pigeon Peas
Polenta
Polydextrose
Polyethylene Glycol
Polyglycerol
Polysorbates
Polysorbate 60
Polysorbate 80
Potassium Benzoate
Potassium Caseinate
Potassium Citrate
Potassium Iodide
Potassium Lactate
Potassium Matabisulphite
Potassium Sorbate
Potatoes
Potato Flour
Potato Starch

Povidone
Prinus
Pristane
Propolis
Propylene Glycol
Propylene Glycol Monosterate
Propyl Gallate
Protease
Psyllium
Pyridoxine Hydrochloride

## Gluten-Free Food Additives

## Q
Quinoa

## R
Ragi
Raisin Vinegar
Rape
Recaldent
Reduced Iron
Rennet
Rennet Casein
Resinous Glaze
Reticulin
Riboflavin
Rice
Rice (Enriched)
Rice Flour
Rice Starch
Rice Syrup
Rice Vinegar
Ricinoleic Acid
Romano Bean (chickpea)
Rosematta
Rosin
Royal Jelly

## Gluten-Free Food Additives

# S

Saccharin
Saffron
Sago
Sago Palm
Sago Flour
Sago Starch
Saifun (bean threads)
Salt
Seaweed
Seeds (except wheat, rye & barley)
Seed - Sesame
Seed - Sunflower
Shea
Sherry Vinegar
Silicon Dioxide
Soba (be sure its 100% buckwheat)
Sodium Acid Pyrophosphate
Sodium Acetate
Sodium Alginate
Sodium Ascorbate
Sodium Benzoate
Sodium Caseinate
Sodium Citrate
Sodium Erythrobate
Sodium Hexametaphosphate
Sodium Lactate
Sodium Lauryl Sulfate
Sodium Metabisulphite
Sodium Nitrate
Sodium Phosphate
Sodium Polyphosphate
Sodium Silaco Aluminate
Sodium Stearoyl Lactylate
Sodium Sulphite
Sodium Stannate
Sodium Tripolyphosphate

Sorbic Acid
Sorbitan Monostearate
Sorbitol-Mannitol (can cause IBS symptoms)
Sorghum
Sorghum Flour
Soy
Soybean
Soy Lecithin
Soy Protein
Soy Protein Isolate
Spices (pure)
Spirits (Specific Types-Identify the grain source)
Spirit Vinegar
Stearates
Stearamide
Stearamine
Stearic Acid
Stearyl Lactate
Stevia
Subflower Seed
Succotash (corn and beans)
Sucralose
Sucrose
Sulfosuccinate
Sulfites
Sulfur Dioxide
Sweet Chestnut Flour

## Gluten-Free Food Additives

# T

Tagatose
Tallow
Tapioca
Tapioca Flour
Tapioca Starch
Tara Gum

Taro
Tarro
Tarrow Root
Tartaric Acid
Tartrazine
TBHQ is Tetra or Tributylhydroquinone
Tea
Tea-Tree Oil
Teff
Teff Flour
Tepary Bean
Textured Vegetable Protein
Thiamin Hydrochloride
Thiamine Mononitrate
Thiamine Hydrochloride
Titanium Dioxide
Tofu (Soy Curd)
Tolu Balsam
Torula Yeast
Tragacanth
Tragacanth Gum
Triacetin
Tricalcium Phosphate
Tri-Calcium Phosphate
Trypsin
Turmeric (Kurkuma)
TVP
Tyrosine

## Gluten-Free Food Additives

# U

Urad/Urid Beans
Urad/Urid Dal (peas) Vegetables
Urad/Urid flour
Urd

## Gluten-Free Food Additives

# V

Vinegar (All except Malt)
Vanilla Extract
Vanilla Flavoring
Vanillin
Vinegars (Specific Types)
Vitamin A (retinol)
Vitamin A Palmitate
Vitamin B1
Vitamin B-12
Vitamin B2
Vitamin B6
Vitamin D
Vitamin E Acetate

## Gluten-Free Food Additives

# W

Waxy Maize
Whey
Whey Protein Concentrate
Whey Protein Isolate
White Vinegar
Wines
Wine Vinegars (& Balsamic)
Wild Rice

# X

Xanthan Gum (replaces "elastic" quality
of gluten)
Xylitol

## Gluten-Free Food Additives

# Y

Yam Flour
Yeast   Yogurt (plain, unflavored)

# Z

Zinc Oxide
Zinc Sulfate

# Gluten-Free Recipes

### 10 inch- Gluten Free Cheese Pizza Recipe

Servings: 4 individual 6-inch pizzas
Ingredients:
* 1 recipe for Gluten Free pizza crust (recipe link below)
* 2 tablespoons good quality olive oil (adds flavor!)
* 1/2 cup good quality pizza sauce (I use Muir Glen Organic Canned Pizza Sauce)
* 2 teaspoons Gluten Free Italian herb blend seasonings OR gluten free dried oregano
* 4 ounces freshly grated provolone cheese
* 1 ounce freshly grated parmesan cheese
* 1 teaspoon crushed red pepper flakes (optional)
Preparation:
Preheat oven to 450° F
If you have a pizza stone place it in oven to preheat. If not, use a baking sheet or round pizza pan.
One recipe of gluten free pizza crust makes about 4 individual 6-inch personal pizzas. (see notes)
* Brush each pizza crust with 1 teaspoon olive oil.
* Evenly spoon 1 heaping tablespoon pizza sauce on each pizza.
* Sprinkle 1 ounce provolone and 1/4 ounce parmesan on each pizza.
* Sprinkle each pizza with about 1/2 teaspoon Italian herbs or oregano. Add crushed red pepper flakes (optional).
* Drizzle about 1/2 teaspoon evenly over cheese layer.
* Bake in preheated oven for about 12 minutes or until cheese is bubbly and crust is golden brown.

Notes- Directions for this recipe are for making 4 small pizzas. If you are making fewer, larger pizzas, adjust ingredients used on each pizza accordingly.

# Gluten Free Tacos with Avocado

6 Servings
Ingredients:
* 6 Gluten Free hard taco shells (See tip)
* 1 pound lean ground beef
* 1 tablespoon olive oil
* 2 tablespoons Gluten Free taco seasoning (See tip)
* 3 tablespoons water
* 2 cups loosely packed, finely shredded baby spinach
* ½ cup finely chopped red onions
* ½ cup chopped fresh avocado
* 1 cup shredded mozzarella cheese
Preparation:
Place taco shells on a baking tray and warm in a 350° oven for 5 minutes.
Brown ground beef in olive oil until completely cooked. On low heat, stir in 2 tablespoons of gluten free taco seasonings and 3 tablespoons of water. Simmer for about 3 minutes, stirring occasionally.
Fill each taco shell with a layer of seasoned ground beef, chopped avocado, chopped onion, shredded spinach and top with shredded cheese. Garnish with a thin slice of avocado.
Tips:
Bearitos® brand hard corn taco shells and taco seasoning are gluten free.

# Gluten Free Spaghetti

6 Servings
Ingredients:
* 1 pound lean ground beef
* 1 25-ounce jar Gluten Free spaghetti sauce
* 1 pound package Gluten Free spaghetti
* 2 tablespoons olive oil
* 1 tablespoon freshly chopped basil (optional)
* 3 ounces freshly grated Parmesan cheese
Preparation:

* Cook Gluten Free spaghetti according to package directions. Drain. Coat with olive oil.
* Brown ground beef. Add spaghetti sauce and basil (optional).
* Simmer sauce for about 15 minutes.
* Serve sauce over warm spaghetti sprinkled with fresh grated Parmesan cheese.

## Fast and Easy Overnight Gluten Free Oatmeal

4 Servings
Ingredients:
* 1 cup Gluten Free rolled oats
* 1 cup warm water
* 2 tablespoons lemon juice or plain Gluten Free yogurt
* 1/2 teaspoon salt
* When you are ready to cook soaked oatmeal:
* 1 cup water
* 1/2 cup raisins (optional)
* 1/4 teaspoon cinnamon (optional)
Preparation:
Pour 1 cup warm water, mixed with 2 tablespoons lemon juice or plain GF yogurt in a wide-
mouth 1-quart thermos. Add whole Gluten Free rolled oats and stir. Put the lid on the thermos. If
you don't have a thermos, place the mixture in a glass bowl, cover and let the bowl sit in a warm
location overnight.
In the morning place soaked oatmeal, 1 cup water, salt and raisins (optional) in a medium
saucepan. Cover and cook over low heat for about 3 minutes. Remove from heat, stir in
cinnamon (optional) and let stand for about 5 minutes. Serve plain, with maple syrup, honey or
your favorite sweetener.

## Gluten Free / Dairy Free High Protein "Banilla" Breakfast Smoothie

2 Servings
Ingredients:
* 2 cups unsweetened dairy free milk substitute (I used organic almond milk)
* 2 ounces dairy free protein powder (I used Healthy-N-Fit 100% Egg Protein Vanilla Ice Cream Flavor). If sensitive to eggs, use Jarrow Pure Plant Protein Powder.
* 1 peeled and sliced medium frozen banana
* 1 teaspoon vanilla extract
* Dash of nutmeg (optional)
Preparation:
Pour 2 cups of chilled rice milk in blender. Add egg white protein powder, frozen banana slices,
vanilla and blend on high until smooth and creamy. Serve garnished with a dash of nutmeg
(optional).
Reminder: Always make sure your work surfaces, utensils, pans and tools are free of gluten.
Always read product labels. Manufacturers can change product formulations without notice.
When in doubt, do not buy or use a product before contacting the manufacturer for verification
that the product is free of gluten.

## Gluten Free Halibut Shrimp Ceviche

Serves 4 to 6
Ingredients:
* 1/2 pound fresh skinless halibut filet, cut into 1/2-inch cubes
* 1/2 pound peeled and deveined shrimp, cut into 1/2-inch cubes
* 1-1/2 cups fresh squeezed lime juice
* 1 medium chopped sweet yellow onion
* 4 sliced green onions
* 3 Roma tomatoes, seeded and chopped into 1/4-inch pieces

* 2 to 3 fresh jalapeno peppers, seeded and finely chopped
* 1/2 cup chopped fresh chopped cilantro, plus extra whole leaves for garnish
* 1/3 cup chopped fresh chopped flat leave parsley
* 4 tablespoons olive oil
* 1/4 cup fresh orange juice or fresh lemon juice
* 2 teaspoons cane sugar, optional
* Salt and pepper to taste
* Serve with Gluten Free corn chips or crackers

Preparation:

Marinade fish and shrimp: Put chopped halibut, shrimp and yellow onion in a 1-1/2 quart glass
bowl. Pour lime juice over all making sure that the juice completely covers all ingredients. If not,
add more lime juice. Cover the bowl and place in refrigerator for about 4 hours.

Check to see if the fish is thoroughly cooked by cutting a piece of halibut in half. If it is opaque,
it's done. If it is still partially translucent in color, put the bowl back in the refrigerator for
another hour and check again. When the halibut is cooked, transfer the mixture to a colander or
mesh strainer and drain off the juice.

In a large bowl combine green onions, tomatoes, jalapeno peppers, cilantro, parsley and olive oil,
orange juice and sugar (if using.)

Gently fold in halibut, shrimp and onion mixture. Season to taste with salt and pepper. If you
prefer a sweeter taste, add more orange juice or sugar as necessary. Cover and Refrigerate until
ready to serve.

Ceviche can be prepared up to two days before serving. Store in tightly covered bowl in the
refrigerator.

Serve with Gluten Free corn chips or crackers.

## Gluten Free Turkey Gravy

Yields: About 2 cups of gravy
Ingredients:
* Reserved pan juices from turkey roasting pan
* 2 tablespoons cornstarch
* 1/2 water OR white wine
* Salt and pepper to taste
Preparation:
When roasted turkey is done cooking, pour pan juices into a 2-cup measuring cup or bowl. Use a
spatula to scrape flavorful pan dripping into the cup or bowl.
When fat rises to the top of the cup, skim off 1/4 cup of fat and pour in a medium skillet or
saucepan. Discard any remaining fat. Mix cornstarch with 1/2 cup water or white wine. Stir until
smooth and dissolved.
Add remaining pan juices to fat in the skillet. Whisk dissolved cornstarch into the pan and cook
over medium heat while continuing to whisk for about 5 minutes, until thickened. Add salt and
pepper to taste.

## Gluten Free Cornbread Dressing

Ingredients:
* 2 cups dry Gluten Free cornbread crumbs
* 2 cups dry Gluten Free bread crumbs
* 1 cup finely chopped celery with leafy tops
* 1 cup sliced green onions (about 8 green onions)
* 2 minced cloves garlic
* 1/4 cup olive oil
* 1/4 cup butter
* 1-2 tablespoons Gluten Free savory herb blend OR poultry herb blend (see tips)
* 3/4 - 1 cup Gluten Free chicken or turkey stock
* Salt and pepper to taste

Preparation:
1. In a large saucepan, melt butter and add olive oil.
2. Add celery, onions and garlic and saute until vegetables are tender, about 5 minutes.
3. Add bread crumbs, salt, pepper and dry herb blend.
4. Pour poultry stock in. Stir to blend. Adjust seasonings and slowly add more stock if necessary.
5. Heat through and serve.

**Gluten Free breads used in this recipe-**
Gluten Free Skillet Cornbread with Apples and Thyme
Gluten Free Walnut Rosemary Bread
**Gluten Free Herb Sources-**
Tone's / Durkee / Spice Island

## Gluten Free Pumpkin Caramel Flan

Yield: 8 to 10 servings
Ingredients:
* Flan Caramel:
* 1/4 cup water
* 3/4 cup pure cane sugar, preferably organic
* Pumpkin Custard Filling:
* 1 cup half-and-half OR 1 cup canned coconut milk (full fat for best results)
* 1 cup heavy cream
* 3/4 cup pure cane sugar, preferably organic
* 1 cup solid pack pumpkin (not sweetened canned pumpkin pie mix)
* 6 large eggs
* 1 teaspoon ground cinnamon
* 1/4 teaspoon ground ginger
* 1/4 teaspoon ground nutmeg
* 1/8 teaspoon ground cloves
* 2 teaspoons vanilla extract
* 1/8 teaspoon salt
Preparation:
Preheat oven to 350° F / 176° C
Have ready a 9-inch round deep dish pie plate and a shallow roasting pan that the pie plate fits in.

Combine water and 3/4 cup sugar in a small heavy saucepan. Heat to boiling. Reduce heat, tilt
pan several times but don't stir. Reduce heat and simmer for 5 to 10 minutes, until mixture turns
a medium amber color. Watch closely to prevent burning. Immediately pour the hot mixture into
pie plate and carefully tilt the plate to evenly coat the bottom of the plate before the sugar
hardens. Set aside.
Combine half-and-half OR coconut milk, heavy cream and 3/4 cup cane sugar in a heavy
saucepan. Heat on medium until warm and sugar dissolves.
Combine pumpkin, eggs, spices, vanilla and salt in a large mixing bowl. Beat on high until
blended.
Slowly drizzle warm cream mixture into pumpkin mixture, whisking until smooth and combined.
Pour pumpkin mixture over the hardened caramelized sugar in pie plate. Place pie plate in
roasting pan and add about 1 1/2 inches of boiling water to roasting pan. Carefully place pan in
preheated oven and bake for 60-70 minutes or just until custard sets. Cool completely and refrigerate until ready to serve. Use a knife to loosen flan from sides of pie
plate. Invert on a plate to serve. Can be prepared and refrigerated up to 2 days before serving.

## Cranberry-Pecan Quinoa Salad

Makes 4 side servings, 2 as a main dish
Ingredients
1/2 cup quinoa, rinsed
3/4 cup water
1/4 cup Craisins
1/4 cup chopped pecans
1 tbsp minced fresh basil
1 tbsp balsamic vinegar
2 tbsp olive oil
Salt
Pepper

Garlic powder

Steps

1. Combine the quinoa and water in a pot, bring to a boil, reduce heat to a simmer, cover, and
cook for 15 minutes. Then remove from heat, remove the lid, and fluff.
2. Add the chopped pecans, Craisins, and basil.
3. In a separate bowl, combine the balsamic vinegar and olive oil. Add a dash each of salt,
pepper, and garlic powder. Mix well.
4. Add the vinaigrette to the quinoa salad and toss to mix. Serve warm or cold.

Notes

To make a cold version of the salad, you could cook the quinoa ahead of time and chill it in the
fridge, then proceed with the remaining steps of the recipe.

## Chicken Cacciatore

Makes 3 servings

Ingredients

1 tbsp olive oil
1 tbsp butter
6 chicken thighs, trimmed of most fat
1/4 cup Artisan Gluten Free Flour Blend
Salt and pepper
4 garlic cloves, minced
1 red bell pepper, diced
1 yellow onion, diced
1/2 cup white wine (such as pinot grigio)
1 1/2 cups diced tomatoes with liquid (one 14.5-ounce can)
1 cup GF chickenbroth
1 tsp dried oregano
1/2 tsp dried rosemary pulsed in a spice grinder
1 bay leaf
2 tbsp nonpareilles capers
2 tbsp chopped fresh basil

Steps

1. In a bowl, season the flour with some salt and pepper. Heat the olive oil and butter in a skillet

over medium-high heat. Dredge the chicken thighs in the flour and cook about 5 minutes per
side, to lightly brown the chicken and cook most of the way. Remove the chicken.

2. Add the garlic to the pan and saute until fragrant, about 30 seconds.

3. Add the pepper and onion and saute until soft, about 4 minutes.

4. Add the white wine and simmer, about 4 more minutes.

5. Add the chicken broth, tomatoes, and dried herbs (oregano, rosemary, bay leaf) and bring to a
simmer.

6. Add the capers and chicken, reduce the heat to medium, and cook the chicken until done,
about 10 minutes.

7. Remove the bay leaf. Garnish with fresh basil. Serve with rice.

Notes

Though we used our signature flour blend to dredge the chicken, you could substitute most any
GF flour or flour blend to do the job.

## Sweet Potato - Black Bean Chili

Makes 6-8 servings
Ingredients
Olive oil
1 medium yellow onion, diced
1 sweet potato (~11 ounces), peeled and diced large
3 14.5-oz cans diced tomatoes, no salt added
1/2 lb black beans, soaked and cooked
3 cups GF chicken broth
1 tsp garlic powder
1 tsp ground cumin
1 tsp ground coriander
1/2 tsp ancho chile powder
1/2 tsp chipotle powder
Juice of 1/2 lime
Cilantro (for garnish)
Steps
1. Heat about 1 tbsp or so of olive oil in a large saucepan. Then saute the onions until soft.

2. Add the sweet potatoes, and saute an additional 5 minutes.
3. Add the remaining ingredients through and including the chipotle powder (but not the lime
and cilantro).
4. Bring to a simmer. Cook about 30 minutes, until the sweet potatoes are soft and the chili's
flavors are well developed.
5. Leave the chili chunky. Or, to prepare as we photographed the dish, reserve about 3/4 cup of
the chili. Puree the remainder with an immersion blender to make a smooth, thick soup.
6. Mix in the lime juice.
7. Add back in the reserved chunky chili (for both texture and presentation). Garnish with fresh,
chopped cilantro.
8. Serve with fresh Gluten Free cornbread.

Notes
For the black beans, we soaked the beans in water overnight. The next day, we drained the water
and rinsed the beans. Then we added new water, and cooked the beans for 1 to 2 hours until
tender. Drain the beans, and they're ready to be used in the recipe!

## Orange-Herb Chicken

Makes 3 servings
Ingredients
3 chicken breasts (boneless, skinless)
1/4 cup Artisan Gluten Free Flour Blend (or any all-purpose GF flour)
Salt and pepper
4 tbsp butter
1 tbsp olive oil
1 tsp Herbs de Provence
1/2 cup orange juice
2 tsp cornstarch
1 cup GF chicken stock

Steps

1. Use a meat mallet (or rolling pin) to flatten the chicken breasts between two pieces of plastic
 wrap.
2. Season the flour with salt and pepper, and dredge the chicken in the flour.
3. Melt 1 tbsp of the butter and the olive oil in a large skillet over medium-high heat. Add the
chicken (in batches, if necessary) and cook 5 minutes per side, or until done. Remove the
chicken from the pan.
4. Add the remaining 3 tbsp butter and the herbs to the pan.
5. Whisk the cornstarch into the orange juice until dissolved fully. Then add the orange juice and
the chicken stock to the pan.
6. Bring to a simmer and cook 5 to 8 minutes, stirring regularly, until the sauce reaches a desired
thickness. Season to taste with salt and pepper.
7. Return the chicken to the pan and toss in the sauce to coat.
Notes
For this recipe, we lightly pounded the chicken breasts, but didn't pound them flat into a true thin
paillard. Either way will work. Just make sure you cook the chicken through fully!

## Gluten Free Granola Bars

36 Servings
Ingredients
* 1 cup corn syrup
* 3/4 cup natural peanut butter
* 1 cup Gluten Free chocolate chips, divided
* 1/2 cup chopped almonds
* 1/2 cup chopped cashews
* 2 cups Gluten Free oatmeal
* 2 cups crispy rice cereal
* 1/3 cup flax seed meal
Directions
1. Mix syrup and peanut butter in a saucepan over low heat until smooth, 3 to 5 minutes.

2. Remove saucepan from heat. Stir about half the chocolate chips into the syrup mixture.
3. Mix remaining chocolate chips, almonds, cashews, oatmeal, crispy rice cereal, and flax seed
meal in a bowl.
4. Pour the mixture from the saucepan over the mixture in the bowl; stir to evenly coat.
5. Transfer mixture to a 9x13-inch baking dish and press into an even layer; allow to cool
completely before cutting into bars.

## Chicken Vesuvio

Makes 4 servings
Ingredients
For the chicken
4 chicken breasts, flattened
1/4 cup Artisan Gluten Free Flour Blend
Salt
Pepper
Dried oregano
Garlic powder
1 tbsp olive oil
1 tbsp butter
For the sauce
1 cup GF chicken broth
1 cup white wine (such as Pinot Grigio)
1 tsp garlic powder
1 tsp dried oregano
2 tbsp butter
For the potatoes
2 large Russet potatoes
Olive oil
Salt
Lemon juice
Dried oregano
Garlic powder
Steps
To make the potatoes:
1. Preheat your oven or toaster oven to 400 deg F.

2. Cut each large Russet potato into 6 long wedges and place in a baking tray.

3. Coat the wedges in olive oil and arrange them so they are wedge-side up.

4. Sprinkle lightly with salt, then a dash of lemon juice, then lightly with dried oregano and
garlic powder.

5. Roast for 45 min to 1 hour, until golden brown and soft.

To cook the chicken:

6. Meanwhile, in a bowl, season the flour with some salt, pepper, dried oregano, and garlic
powder (about 1/2 tsp of each). Heat the olive oil and butter in a skillet over medium-high heat.
Dredge the chicken breasts in the flour and cook about 5 minutes per side, to lightly brown the
chicken and cook through. Remove the chicken. (If necessary, cook the chicken in batches,
depending on the size of your skillet.)

To make the sauce:

7. Add the chicken broth, white wine, garlic, and oregano to a skillet. Bring to a boil over high
heat and reduce the sauce for 10 minutes.

8. Add the butter, turn the heat down to medium, and cook for 2 more minutes.

9. Remove from the heat and add back the chicken.

To finish the dish:

10. Plate 1 chicken breast and 3 potato wedges per serving. Garnish with green peas.

Notes

For the flour dredge, you can use most any Gluten Free flour or all-purpose GF blend.

For a saucier version, double the sauce quantities.

# Gluten Free Granola

12 servings
2 cups puffed rice
2 cups puffed corn
1 cup Perky's Nutty Rice cereal
1 cup Kashi Cranberry Sunshine cereal
1 cup roasted peanuts
2 teaspoons vanilla
1/2 cup honey
1/2 cup light corn syrup
1/4 cup vegetable oil
1/2 cup raisins
1/2 cup dried cranberries
nonstick spray
1. Preheat the oven to 250 degrees.
2. In a large bowl, combine the puffed rice, puffed corn, Perky's Nutty Rice Cereal, Kashi
Cranberry Sunshine cereal, peanuts, vanilla extract, honey, and light corn syrup.
3. In a small saucepan, heat the honey and oil over medium heat (it just needs to get warm so it
flows easier; don't overheat).
4. Pour the warm honey and oil over mixed ingredients.
5. Place the mixture (you haven't added the fruit yet) onto large baking sheets that have been
coated with cooking spray.
6. Bake the granola for 2 hours, stirring every 15 minutes to keep the mixture from sticking.
7. Carefully add the raisins and cranberries to the hot granola and serve.
Tip: Homemade granola tends to go stale quickly. Extend the life of your homemade granola by
using a vacuum-packing system to seal and store several individual-sized servings. Too late? If
your granola has already gone stale, use it to make granola bars.

## Rosemary Shrimp Skewers with Arugula-White Bean Salad

Ingredients
3 tablespoons plus 1 teaspoon extra virgin olive oil
3 tablespoons plus 2 teaspoons fresh lemon juice
3 garlic cloves, smashed
2 teaspoons minced fresh rosemary
3/4 teaspoon salt
1/4 teaspoon plus 1/8 teaspoon black pepper
1 1/2 pounds extra-large shrimp, shelled and cleaned, tails on
Nonstick cooking spray
1 small garlic clove, minced
Pinch sugar
1 5-ounce package baby arugula
1 15-ounce can cannellini beans, rinsed and drained
1/2 small red onion, thinly sliced
Directions
1. Combine 2 tablespoons of the olive oil, 1 tablespoon of the lemon juice, the smashed garlic
cloves, the rosemary, 1/2 teaspoon of the salt, and 1/4 teaspoon of the black pepper in a medium
bowl. Add the shrimp; toss well. Cover and refrigerate 15 minutes.
2. Heat a grill to medium-high. Thread shrimp on skewers (if they're wooden, soak in water 30
minutes prior to grilling) and discard marinade. Lightly mist grill with cooking spray. Grill
shrimp until just cooked through, about 2 minutes per side.
3. Combine the minced garlic, sugar, and remaining olive oil, lemon juice, salt, and black pepper
in a large bowl. Add the arugula, beans, and onion; toss to combine.
4. Mound the salad on one side of a large platter and arrange the shrimp skewers alongside.

## Gluten-Free Shopping Reminders

Enjoy all fresh (preferably organic) fruits, vegetables, nuts, wild caught fish, shellfish, and grass-
fed meats as long as they are not processed (ie., mixes, sauces, canned, meals). Evaluate
ingredient labels whenever evaluating a processed food.
Oats are gluten-free, but may be grown or processed with wheat during. This contamination
leaves oats as a questionable item. Look for oat products that are gluten-free.
The list below is not all inclusive, but includes popular food items. When in doubt, put it back
on the shelf and do your research.

## Gluten-Free Food Lists - Grains, Dairy, Meats/Fish
## Grains

Amaranth
Buckwheat
Corn
Millet
Montina (Indian rice grass)
Oats** opt for a Gluten-Free product
Quinoa
Rice
Sorghum
Teff
Wild Rice
**Dairy (always check labels)**
Check for lactose intolerance
Organic is always preferred
Plain milk, but avoid flavored milk (substitute almond milk if lactose intolerant)
Plain yogurt is usually safe, check flavored yogurts
Eggs
Butter
Cottage Cheese

Ice Cream and Sherberts proceed with caution
Non-processed cheese, but watch out for "beer washed" cheeses
Meats, Fish, Shellfish, Nuts
All non-processed, otherwise check additive list and ingredients.
Grass-fed organic meats and nuts and wild caught fish preferred.

# Helpful and Trusted Resources

**American Autoimmune Related Diseases Association, Inc.**
Dedicated to eradicating auto-immune diseases through patient education, auto-immune disease research, public awareness, and advocacy as well as patient services.

**www.aarda.org**

**Celiac Disease Foundation**
Celiac Disease Foundation is a non-profit, public benefit corporation dedicated to providing services and support regarding celiac disease and dermatitis herpetiformis, through programs of awareness, education, advocacy and research.

**http://celiac.org/**

**The Celiac Disease Foundation's Gluten-Free Resource Directory**
Unique and easy, one-stop guide to all things Gluten-Free

**http://cdfresourcedirectory.com/**

**U.S. Department Of Health And Human Services**
National Digestive Diseases Information Clearinghouse (NDDIC)

Information on celiac disease in Spanish

Lo que usted debe saber sobre la enfermedad celíaca

**http://digestive.niddk.nih.gov/spanish/pubs/celiac_ez/index.aspx**

**The University of Chicago Celiac Disease Center**
Celiac Disease Facts and Figures
**http://www.uchospitals.edu/pdf/uch_007937.pdf**

**Celiac Disease and Gluten-free Diet Information Since 1995**
Celiac disease and gluten-free diet information at Celiac.com. Celiac disease, also known as gluten intolerance, is a genetic disorder that affects at least 1 in 133 Americans. Symptoms of celiac disease can range from the classic features, such as diarrhea, weight loss, and malnutrition, to latent symptoms such as isolated nutrient deficiencies but no gastrointestinal symptoms.
**http://celiac.com**

**The Gluten Free Diet Review**
The Gluten-Free Diet: How to Provide Effective Education and Resources
**http://internal.medicine.ufl.edu/files/2012/07/5.18.03.01.-Gluten-Free-Diet-review.pdf**

**Research in Autism Spectrum Disorders**
Gluten-free and casein-free diets in the treatment of autism spectrum disorders: A systematic review
**http://www.edb.utexas.edu/education/assets/files/ltc/gfcf_review.pdf**

**National Foundation for Celiac Awareness**
Through empowerment, education and advocacy, the National Foundation for Celiac Awareness (NFCA) drives diagnoses of celiac disease and other gluten-related disorders and improves the quality of life for those on a lifelong gluten-free diet.
**http://www.celiaccentral.org/**

**Coeliac Australia**
Coeliac Australia's Vision is to enhance the quality of life of people requiring a gluten free diet for life and to encourage and support research towards a cure or other ethical forms of treatment for coeliac disease.
**http://www.coeliac.org.au/**

Gluten Intolerance Group of North America – GIG
**The Gluten Intolerance Group (GIG) is an organization for supporting patients living with from**

gluten-sensitive diseases (celiac disease, dermatitis herpetiformis, and gluten intolerances), in
order to live health lives. The Group is administered by health care professionals who are able to
advise its members on diet. The Group holds provides education materials at no charge from its
Web site and holds events such as education conferences.
www.gluten.net/

## Check out other products offered by Path to Health and Healing at:

http://www.pathtohealthandhealing.com/products/

- Seeds 4 Change: A Path to Health and Healing (book, online course and audio program)

- Hormonal Roller Coaster (online course)

- High Quality Supplemental Support at
  http://www.purerxo.com/pathtohealthandhealing/rxo/home.asp

www.ingramcontent.com/pod-product-compliance
Lightning Source LLC
Chambersburg PA
CBHW071219280526
45787CB00002B/730